YOUR KNOWLEDGE HAS VALUE

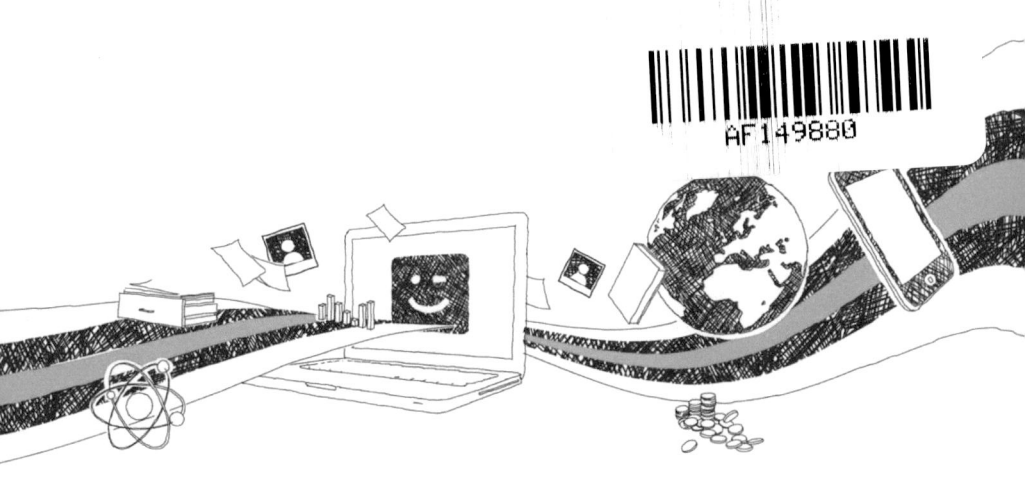
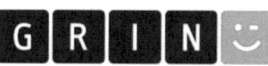

Bibliographic information published by the German National Library:

The German National Library lists this publication in the National Bibliography; detailed bibliographic data are available on the Internet at http://dnb.dnb.de .

Imprint:

Copyright © 2015 GRIN Verlag, Open Publishing GmbH
Print and binding: Books on Demand GmbH, Norderstedt Germany
ISBN: 978-3-668-05540-7

This book at GRIN:

http://www.grin.com/en/e-book/306842/the-effect-of-polymethylmethacrylate-on-dental-modelling-wax

Amer Taqa, Luma M. Al-Nema, Amrah Y. Al-Jmmal

The effect of polymethylmethacrylate on dental modelling wax

GRIN Publishing

GRIN - Your knowledge has value

Since its foundation in 1998, GRIN has specialized in publishing academic texts by students, college teachers and other academics as e-book and printed book. The website www.grin.com is an ideal platform for presenting term papers, final papers, scientific essays, dissertations and specialist books.

Visit us on the internet:

http://www.grin.com/

http://www.facebook.com/grincom

http://www.twitter.com/grin_com

The Effect of recycled polymethylmethacrylate Additive on the physical properties of Dental Modelling Wax

Amer A Taqa[1]*, Luma M. Al-Nema[2], Amrah Y. Al-Jmmal[3]

[2,3]University of Mosul, College of Dentistry, Department of Prosthodontics
[1]*University of Mosul, College of Dentistry, Department of DBS

Abstract

Aim of the study: The aim of this study is to investigate the effect of recycled polymethylmethacrylate particlesaddedat the melting point,hardness, flow and linear thermal expansion properties.

Material and Method: Modeling wax was prepared by mixing 65 grams of paraffin with 30 grams of beeswax. The modeling wax was prepared by melting the ingredients together under continuous stirring at the temperature 45°C in the water bath, after that 20% of recycled polymethyl methacrylate added slowly to mixture at 45°C and rapid mixing together until obtaining a homogenous mixture. Then, the mixtures were poured into the molds and stored at room temperature for 24 hours prior totesting the melting point, flow, hardness and thermal expansion testing.

The results: The value of mean offlow of modeling wax with additive appeared less than control, the degree of mean of flow are about 60% while the mean of control 75%. The fore needle penetration test alsomodeling wax with additive appeared more harder than the control. Themean of linear thermal expansion of modeling wax with additiveis decreased. There is a statistically significant difference at $p \leq 0.05$ between modelling wax with additive and control.

Conclusions: The addition of recycled polymethylmethacrylate particles 20% to bees wax and hard paraffin leads to decrease the flow, thermal expansion and dimensional changes, but increase the melting point and hardness when compared with commercial modelling wax (control).

Keywords: recycle Polymethylmethacrylate Additive, dental wax.

Introduction

Waxes are organic polymers consisting of hydrocarbons and their derivatives (e.g. Esters and alcohols). Waxes used in dentistry may be composed of several ingredients, including natural waxes, synthetic waxes, natural and synthetic resins, and other additions such as oil, fats, gums, fatty acids, and coloring agents of various types[1,2].

The chemical components of both natural and synthetic waxes impart characteristics to the wax, which determines of primary interest since the specific physical properties of a wax its usefulness for the intended application. So, by the blending of appropriate natural and synthetic waxes and resins and other additives, we can achieve the particular characteristics needed for the job at hand of each dental wax[3,4].

The main ingredient of dental waxes is 70% to 80% paraffin, Paraffin is a mixture of solid hydrocarbon, obtained from petroleum, and 20%to 30% beeswax. Beeswax is a substance obtained from bee honeycombs and consists of an ester complex mixture, saturated and unsaturated hydrocarbons, and organic acid with high molecule's weight.This mixture is carried out to produce a material with the required properties for a specific application[5,6].

The utility of dental waxes stems from several factors:they are cheap, non-toxic, low melting, weak solids that canbe readily shaped and molded. They are used in some of thehighest precision work in dentistry[7].While flow is important in every dental wax application,complicated by residual stress effects and thermal expansion, flow results from the slippage of waxmolecules over each other. It is a measure of a wax's ability to deform underlight forces and is analogous to creep. Generally, the rheological principles remain valid in wax systems[8].

Inorganic filler can act as an effective hardener for natural wax blended for dental applications. The addition of inorganic filler up to 10% in paraffin and beeswax blend could increase hardness and decrease melting point.Filler addition in resins and waxes will reduce the plasticity of matrix, increase hardness and reduce thermal expansion[9,10].

Fourier transform infrared spectroscopy(FTIR),is one of the most common spectroscopic techniques used by organic and inorganic chemists. Simply, it is the absorption measurement of different IR frequencies by a sample positioned in the path of an IR beam. The main goal of spectroscopic analysis is to determine the chemical functional groups in the sample[11].

Aim of the study: The aim of this study is to investigate the effect of recycled polymethylmethacrylateparticlesafter addedatthe melting point,hardness,flow and linear thermal expansion properties.

Materials and Method

The materials used in this research were Paraffin (Pertamina, Indonesia), yellow beeswax (North of Iraq),recycled polymethylmethacrylate (China).

Preparation of additive

One gram of recycled polymethylmethacrylateparticlesdissolved in 5 ml of chloroform, then mixed until all particles completely dissolved,to obtain 20% of the additive.

Preparation of materials

Modeling wax was prepared by mixing 65 grams of paraffin with 30 grams of beeswax. The modeling wax was prepared by melting the ingredients together under continuous stirringat 45°C in the water bath, after that 20%of recycled polymethylmethacrylate added slowly to mixture at 45° C and rapid mixing together until obtaining a homogenous mixture.Then, the mixture was poured into the moulds and stored at room temperature for 24 hours prior to testing. The mixture was poured into acylindrical metal mould for hardness specimens (6 mm thickand 10 mm)diameter[20]. Five specimens were made from each composition for each test. Commercial modelingwax(major Parodotti, Italy) was used as a control group.

Fourier transform infrared spectroscopy (FTIR)

To determine the chemical change in the sample,the modelling wax and mixture with additivewas detected by (FTIR)to determine if there is any chemical change occurs as show in (Figure1,2,3), the measurements were done by using the Alfa Bruker instrument. Mosul University, College of Dentistry.

Determine the melting point of modeling wax with additive

The melting point was measured byusing the Electro-thermal melting point apparatus (CE, VWR, International). The capillary tube was filled as follows: about 0.1 gm of wax is inserted through the opened end of capillary tube with gentle tapping of the capillary tube until the material reaches the closed end of the capillary tube. The procedure was repeated until the length of lightly packed material is 3-5 mm. The filled capillary tube is placed inside the Electrothemal melting point apparatus, until the wax starts to melt, the conclusion of this test is shown in (Table1).

Flow Test Determination

Five specimens of modelling wax with additive and control with(6mm thick and10mm) diameter, were made from each composition for each test,the initial height of the specimen is determined at room temperature (20 ± 2)°C using Electronic digital caliper. Four measurements are made around the circumference and one measurement is made in the center of the specimen. The flow testing instrument and wax specimen were placed in a water bath and held at testing temperature for 20 min. A Constant axial load of 19.6 N (2kg) force was then applied to the specimen for 10 min, after which the specimen, then removed and cooled in air at room temperature and the final height is determined in the same manner as the original height, the flow evidenced by the change in height and reported as percentage of the total height,as shown in(Figure4).

Hardnesstest (Needle Penetration Test)

Hardness was at room temperature (ISO/DIS 1561, 1994), a sample (6 mm) thick and (10 mm) diameter, cylindrical in shape was used. In this test, the standard Vicat apparatus is used. Needle of specified dimension (1mm) and mass (300gm) was to be held vertically against the surface of the wax specimen and released, after (5 ± 0.1) second the needle is stopped; the vertical travel defining the penetrative (flow).The depth of penetration is measured by Electronic digital caliper at room temperature (20 ± 2)°C. Four measurements are made around the circumference and one measurement is made in the center of the specimen. Then, the mean of five measurements was calculated for each.

2

Linear Thermal Expansion: (ADA specification No. 24, 2003)

The five specimens were heated to 25°C and 40°C and the distance between the reference marks at the lower temperature and the change in length on heating to higher temperature is determined.The wax specimen is placed under the holder as shown in (Figure 4) and the reference marks pass through the openings of the holder.The distance between the reference marks is determined to the nearest 0.01 mm. The electronic digital caliper is used to make the measurement. An initial measurement is made in water after 20 min at (25± 0.1) °C. The 25°C temperature was used as zero point. The temperature is then raised in water bath to (40± 0.1) °C. The specimen remains 20 min at that temperature before the distance between reference marks is determined. Three measurements for each sample were obtained and the mean of these measurements was calculated.The change in length was measured and the thermal expansion is calculated as percentage of the total length of the specimen.

Results

The value of mean of modelling wax with additive and control and Multiple analysis range test for flow test, needle penetration test and linear thermal expansion are shown in Figure (5).So modelling wax with the additiveprovided more flow than control, the degreeof mean flow is about 60% whilethe mean of control 75%. The Fore needle penetration test also modelling wax with additive appeared more harder than the control.For linear thermal expansion,mean of modelling wax with additiveis about (0.12 mm) while mean of control (0.22 mm).There is a statistically significant difference at $p \leq 0.05$ between modelling wax with additive and controlas shownin Table (2). The Ftir spectra showed that when added the recycled poly methyl methacrylate particles, the result showed from both charts there is no any chemical change occurs in this material as shown in (Figure 3), the two charts while physical change occurred.

Disscusion

In general, filler materials are added to certain composition in purpose to increase the hardness of mixture, increase toughness, quality, avoids bubbles, decrease flow and thermal expansion, smoother carving, improve accuracy, and free of tackiness to models and instruments[9].

Melting point of Modelling wax with additive

The filler addition up to 10% prohibit the melting properties of wax mixtures. Based on that research, the higher temperature was needed in the melting of wax mixtures with filler. The inorganic filler particles in wax mixtures had functioned as seeds to form a gel structure. The energy that was accepted by thewax was absorbed by the gel structure of filler particles, so the amount of heat absorbed by paraffin wax was decreased. This caused the increasing of wax melting point[12],this agree with the result of this study.

The FTIR spectra it is possible to see a clear wax and wax containing recycling polymer(figure1) wax paraffin contains hydrocarbons only with C-H and C-C bonds. In figure 1, FTIR spectra of paraffin C- H stretching vibrations of saturated hydrocarbons are seen below 3000 cm^{-1}, -CH$_3$ and C-H deformations at about 1472 cm^{-1} and 1377 cm^{-1}. Rocking and wagging of -CH$_2$- gives a clear peak at 719cm^{-1}. Figure 2,3 showed the polymer after incorporated with the wax not lead to change any chemical reactions of wax but work as a mixture material. The identical of the two charts confirm this suggestion. When comparison between the two charts (figur3) it is clear showed there are bands in the 1507,1540 and 1653 cm^{-1} region not found in the spectra of wax alone, because these bands refer to the poly methymathacrylate.

Flow test

The incorporated filler particles reduced the flow of the natural waxes, especially of the ester-containing beeswax, and improved the elastic modulus and strength. A Good correlation was found between the ingredient proportions and measured properties, the experimental blends exhibited properties that are potentially useful for a range of clinical applications[13].

Morgan studied the mechanical properties of beeswax and measured these properties as a function of temperature. They used a variety of techniques and compared them with each other. In their study, the coefficient of friction of beeswax was measured and compared with that of plastic and Nylon 66. They found that the frictional behavior of beeswax departs from Amontons' laws and behaves instead as a classic soft, elastic polymer[14]. The physical and mechanical properties determined in this study include the density and uniaxial compressive strength for beeswax and paraffin wax samples by comparison of the stress-strain relationship between beeswax and paraffin wax to simulate the behavior of reservoir rock in the field[15].Revealed that there was a significant reduction in the flow of hard paraffin at 40°C and 45°C with the addition of 10% and 20% beeswax as in experimental modelling waxes so,the flow reduced more by increasing the percentage of addition from 10% to 20% and this is in agreement with our result[16].

Hardness test (Needle Penetration Test) and Linear Thermal Expansion

The penetration depth of control andadditive wax were in the range of(0.73,0.58)mm respectively. The higher filler concentration showed the increasing of additivewax hardness, that expressed by lower penetration depth. The hardness value of the group without filler was lower than the additive wax.Numerous natural resins are blended with waxes to develop waxes for dental applications. They are compatible with most natural waxes and produce harder products[7]. The new prepared modeling wax with additive showed nearly the same measurement penetration test of Major Parodotti Dentari (Italy)[17].

The results were similar to previous studies on series of filler content of composite restorative materials that showed the filler influence with strong positive correlation on the elastic properties[18].Silica as inorganic filler effectively played important role in the increasing of wax mixture hardness.The linear thermal expansion of carving waxes was in variation, but lower than the inlay wax product (GC, Japan). Those values were also lower than the typical inlay wax,paraffin wax structure consists of covalent bonds with the non-polar coordination. The non-polar bond with other molecules had weakness properties, making the other molecules moved easily. The smaller the amount of non-polar bond in the compound caused the smaller the expansion when the material was heated.In general, the filler was mixed in physico-chemically with wax while decreasing the paraffin volume. This phenomenon caused the decreasing of expansion in heating and contraction in cooling of carving wax[19], this agrees with our result.The addition of 10% and 20% beeswax to hard paraffin led to a significant increase in the hardness of paraffin wax and made it less brittle as in experimental modelling waxes. This is attributed to the effect of beeswax that leads to increase the melting temperature of the mixture and increasing hardness and reduce the flow at room temperature[16], this is agreeing with our result.

Widjijonowas concluded that serums was with high ca-bentolite filter composition had a high melting pointand hardness,but low linear thermal expansion[20].

The modification of dental wax was improving the physical properties than the commercial one. The high percentage of beeswax improves the hardness and thermal coefficient in comparing to commercial wax. The presence of paraffin wax improves the melting range of wax[21].

Conclusions

The addition of recycled polymethylmethacrylateparticles 20% to beeswax and hard paraffin leads to decrease the flow, thermal expansion and dimensional changes, but increase the melting point and hardness when compared with commercial modelling wax (control).

References

[1]. 1.O' Brien W. J. (2002) Dental Materials and Their Selection 3th Ed Quintessenz Publishing Co.Inc.
[2]. 2.Ohnmacht, P., Hasert, G. and Schneiderbanger, T. (2001) Dentale Wachse Quintessenz Zahntech 27, 63-74.
[3]. 3.Hossain, M.E., An Experimental and Numerical Investigation of Memory-Based Complex Rheology and Rock/Fluid Interactions, PhD dissertation, Dalhousie University, Halifax, Nova Scotia, Canada, 2008, p. 773.
[4]. 4.Hossain, M.E., Ketata, C. and Islam, M.R, A Comparative Study of Physical and Mechanical Properties of Natural and Synthetic Waxes for Developing Models for Drilling Applications, Journal of Characterization and Development of Novel Materials, Vol. 1(3), 2009, in press.
[5]. Departemen Kehutanan. Perlebahandi Indonesia. 2005. Available at: http://www/ dephut.go.id /informasi/HUMAS/lebah.htm. Accessed,April 29, 2009.
[6]. Strahl, Pitsch. Beeswax. Available from: http://www.spwax.com. Accessed October 28, 2004.
[7]. Craig RG and Powers JM Restorative Dental Materials. 11th ed., Mosby, (2002): pp. 424-448.
[8]. Darvell B. W. Materials Science for Dentistry 7thed.23 Shawan Drive pokfulam , (2002)University of Hong Kong.
[9]. Anonymous. MDM Corporation expanding dealership, network, inquiries, solicited, Available from: http:/indiamart.com. Accessed February 28, 2007.
[10]. Manappallil JJ. Basic dental materials. 2nd Ed. New Delhi: Jaypee Brothers Medical Pub; 2003. p. 149–50, 276.
[11]. Swann I,Patwardhan S.,Application of Fourier Transform Infrared Spectroscopy (FTIR) forassessing biogenic silica sample purity in geochemical analyses and palaeo enviromental research. Copernicus Publications on behalf of the European GeosciencesUnionClim.Past2011,7,65–74.
[12]. Irnawati D., Pengaruh rasio malam parafin dengan malam carnauba terhadap titik leleh dan kekerasan malam ukir. Laporan Penelitian. FKG–UGM; 2007.

4

[13]. Kotsiomiti E and McCabe J,Experimental wax mixtures for dental use, Journal of OralRehabilitation,2008,Volume 24, Issue 7, pages 517-521.

[14]. Morgan, J., Townley, S., Kemble, G. and Smith, R., Measurement of Physical and Mechanical Properties of Beeswax, Materials Science and Technology, Vol. 18(4), 2002, p. 463–467.

[15]. Enamul M,Chefi K,Rafiqul M, Experimental Study OF Physical AND Mechanical Properties Of Natural and Synthetic Waxes, Using Uniaxial Compressive Strength Test,Proceedings of the Third International Conference on Modeling, Simulation and Applied Optimization Sharjah, 2009.U.A.E January 20-22.

[16]. Alubaidi A., Prosthetic Application of Experimental Modelling Wax with Some Additives,Thesis,College of Dentistry in Mosul University 2008.

[17]. Nadira A,Amer Taqa andWafa M, Preparation and modifying a new type of waxes,2006, Al–RafidainDenJ.2006;6(1):64-71.

[18]. Masouras K, Sikkas N, Watts D. Correlation of filler content and elastic properties of resin-composites. Dental Materials 2008; 24(7):932–39.

[19]. Noort RV. Introduction to dental materials. 3rd edEidenburg: Mosby Elsevier; 2008.p.54–56.

[20]. WidjijonoA.,Agustiono P.,Dyah I, Mechanical properties of carving wax with various Ca-bentolite filter composition,Dental. Journal, 2009 ,Vol. 42. No. 3 .

[21]. Ibtehal H., Nadia T. Jaffer,Mohammed M., Evaluation of some physical properties of prepared molding wax in comparison to commercial available wax.Al–Rafidain DenJ., 2013.

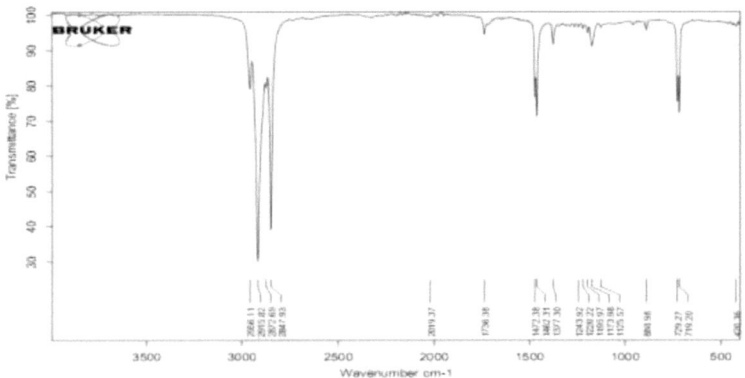

Figure 1: FTIR for the wax alone, own figure

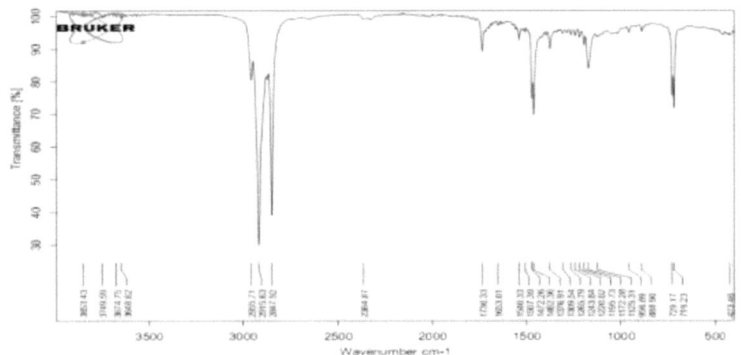

Figure 2: FTIR for the wax with additive, own figure

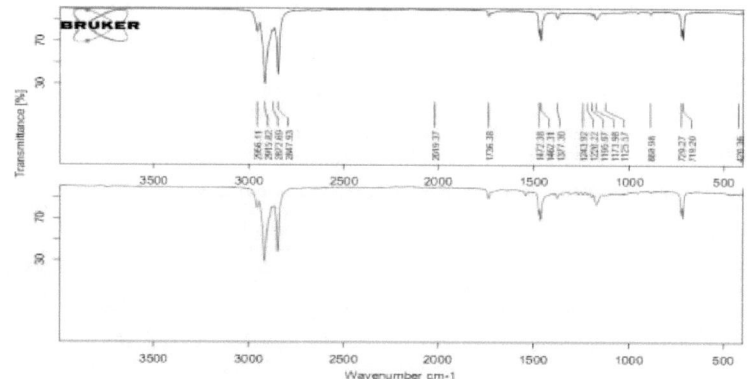

Figure 3: comparative between wax before and after adding, own figure

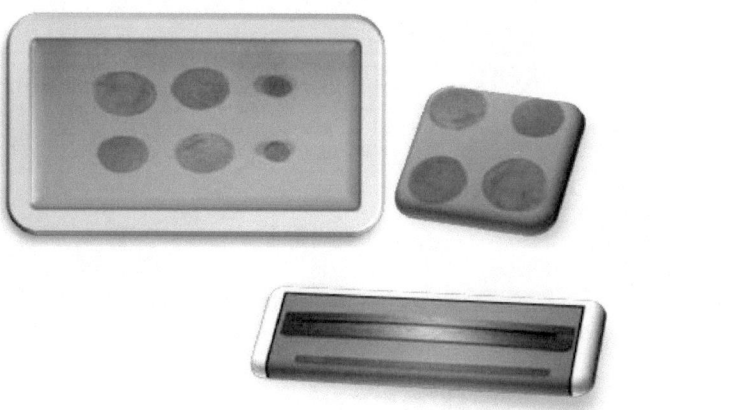

Figure 4 : Samples of flow and thermal expansion test, own figure

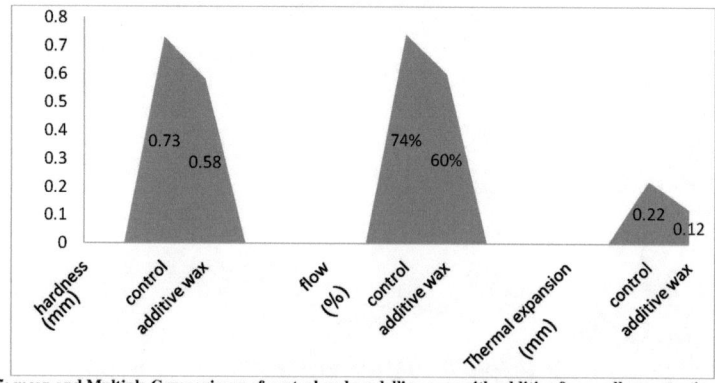

Figure 5: mean and Multiple Comparisons of control and modelling wax with additive for needle penetration test flow test and linear thermal expansion. Own figure.

Table (1): melting point of control and modelling wax with additive, own table.

	Initial time	Final time
Commercial modelling wax(control)	55° C	62° C
Modelling wax with additive	58° C	63° C

Table (2) Independent Samples Test for needle penetration test flow test and linear thermal expansion, own table.

		t-test for Equality of Means			
		T	df	p-value	Mean Difference
Hard	Equal variances assumed	4.254	10	.013	.1466667
Thermal	Equal variances assumed	5.029	10	.007	.0933333
Flow	Equal variances assumed	14.524	10	.000	15.000

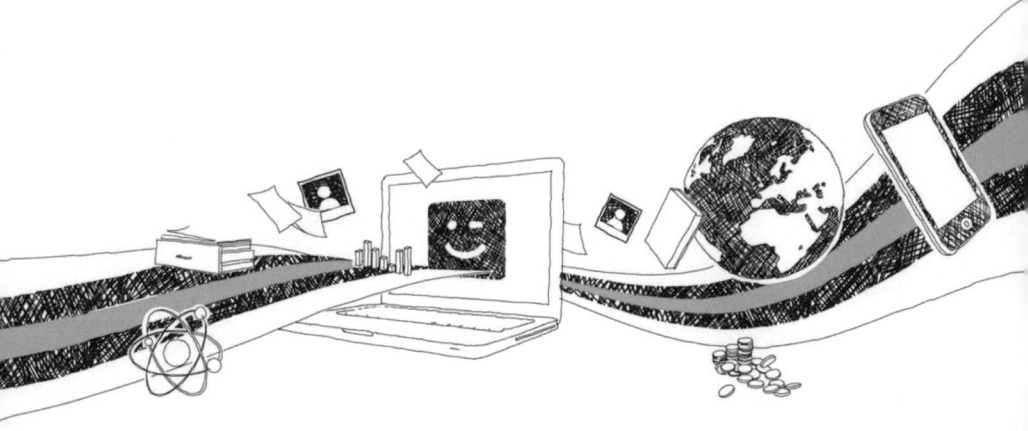
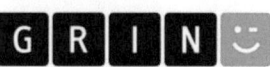